Alkaline Plant Based Diet

A Women's 3-Week Step-by-Step With Recipes and a Meal Plan

mf

copyright © 2020 Stephanie Hinderock

All rights reserved No part of this book may be reproduced, or stored in a retrieval system, or transmitted in any form or by any means, electronic, mechanical, photocopying, recording, or otherwise, without express written permission of the publisher.

Disclaimer

By reading this disclaimer, you are accepting the terms of the disclaimer in full. If you disagree with this disclaimer, please do not read the guide.

All of the content within this guide is provided for informational and educational purposes only, and should not be accepted as independent medical or other professional advice. The author is not a doctor, physician, nurse, mental health provider, or registered nutritionist/dietician. Therefore, using and reading this guide does not establish any form of a physician-patient relationship.

Always consult with a physician or another qualified health provider with any issues or questions you might have regarding any sort of medical condition. Do not ever disregard any qualified professional medical advice or delay seeking that advice because of anything you have read in this guide. The information in this guide is not intended to be any sort of medical advice and should not be used in lieu of any medical advice by a licensed and qualified medical professional.

The information in this guide has been compiled from a variety of known sources. However, the author cannot attest to or guarantee the accuracy of each source and thus should not be held liable for any errors or omissions.

You acknowledge that the publisher of this guide will not be held liable for any loss or damage of any kind incurred as a result of this guide or the reliance on any information provided within this guide. You acknowledge and agree that you assume all risk and responsibility for any action you undertake in response to the information in this guide.

Using this guide does not guarantee any particular result (e.g., weight loss or a cure). By reading this guide, you acknowledge that there are no guarantees to any specific outcome or results you can expect.

All product names, diet plans, or names used in this guide are for identification purposes only and are the property of their respective owners. The use of these names does not imply endorsement. All other trademarks cited herein are the property of their respective owners.

Where applicable, this guide is not intended to be a substitute for the original work of this diet plan and is, at most, a supplement to the original work for this diet plan and never a direct substitute. This guide is a personal expression of the facts of that diet plan.

Where applicable, persons shown in the cover images are stock photography models and the publisher has obtained the rights to use the images through license agreements with third-party stock image companies.

Table of Contents

Introduction 7
Alka-what? 9
   Understanding Alkalinity in Our Body's Internal Environment ... 9
   How Does Diet Work in Our Body? 11
Alkaline Aligns with Women for a Specific Purpose 13
   Osteoporosis 13
   Breast Cancer 14
   Polycystic Ovary Syndrome (PCOS) 14
   Menopause Symptoms 15
   Cardiovascular Disease 15
   Pregnancy Health 16
The Alkaline Plant Based Diet 17
   Principles of Alkaline Plant Based Diet 17
   Benefits of Alkaline Plant Based Diet 18
   Disadvantages of Alkaline Plant Based Diet 19
A 5-Step-by-Step Guide To Getting Started With The Diet 21
   Step 1: Educate Yourself 21
   Step 2: Purge Your Pantry 23
   Step 3: Meal Planning 24
   Step 4: Hydrate Well 26
   Step 5: Track Your Progress 27
   Foods to Eat and to Avoid 29
   Tips on Incorporating These Foods into Daily Meals 30
   Explanation of Why These Foods Are Not Ideal for the Alkaline Diet 31
   Tips on Finding Healthier Alternatives to These Foods 32
Week 1: Heating It Up 34
   What meals do I need to eat? 36
   Do I need to learn how to cook dishes? 36

Week 2: Starting the Engine   **38**

   So, below are some tips on how to face the grocery battlefield: 38

   How do you make a meal plan?   40

7-Day Sample Meal Plan   **42**

Curated Recipes   **46**

   Quinoa Porridge   47

   Chickpea Salad with Lemon-Tahini Dressing   49

   Stuffed Bell Peppers   51

   Green Smoothie   53

   Lentil Soup with a Side of Mixed Greens   54

   Baked Sweet Potato   56

   Chia Seed Pudding with Almond Milk   58

   Quinoa Salad with Roasted Vegetables   59

   Grilled Zucchini and Eggplant Skewers   61

   Vegetable Stir-Fry with Tofu   63

   Lentil and Vegetable Curry served with Quinoa   65

   Spaghetti Squash with Homemade Tomato Sauce   67

   Baked Falafel Salad   69

   Stuffed Portobello Mushrooms with Quinoa and Spinach   71

   Vegan Chili   73

   Green Juice made with Cucumber, Spinach, Apple, and Lemon 75

Conclusion   **76**

FAQ   **79**

References and Helpful Links   **81**

Introduction

Living in a digital age, health and wellness information is abundantly available. Amidst the deluge of dietary advice, one diet plan that has steadily gained recognition over the years is the alkaline plant-based diet. But what sets it apart from other diets? How does it align with your health journey? Let's demystify this together.

The alkaline plant-based diet goes beyond being a fleeting fad; it's a scientifically backed approach to eating, grounded in the concept of maintaining balance in our body's pH levels. This diet advocates for the consumption of foods high in alkaline content - primarily fruits, vegetables, nuts, and legumes - while reducing intake of acidic foods such as meat, dairy, and processed foods.

But it's not about drastic alterations or rigid rules. It's about making informed choices, understanding your body's needs, and slowly integrating healthier foods into your daily meals.

In this guide, we will talk about the following:

- What is Alkaline?

- Understanding Alkalinity in Our Body's Internal Environment
- How Does Diet Work in Our Body?
- Alkaline Aligns with Women for a Specific Purpose
- The Alkaline Plant Based Diet
- A Step-by-step Guide to Getting Started With Alkaline Plant Based Diet
- Foods to Eat and To Avoid
- Sample Meal Plan and Curated Recipes

So, let's take this journey together. Explore the world of the alkaline plant-based diet and discover how it could be a stepping stone towards a healthier, more vibrant version of yourself.

Alka-what?

The term "alkaline" comes from alkali, which refers to the basic, ionized salts in chemistry. In simpler terms, alkalinity is a measure of the ability of a solution to neutralize acids to the equivalence point of carbonate or bicarbonate. The pH scale, ranging from 0 (most acidic) to 14 (most alkaline), is used to determine the acidity or alkalinity of a substance. A pH value of 7 is regarded as neutral, indicating that it's neither on the acidic side nor the alkaline end of the spectrum.

Understanding Alkalinity in Our Body's Internal Environment

Our body strives to maintain a slightly alkaline state, usually around a pH of 7.4, for optimal functioning. This pH balance plays a critical role in our body processes, including metabolism, enzyme function, nutrient absorption, and immune response. When our bodies become too acidic, due to factors like stress, unhealthy diet, or exposure to environmental toxins, it can disrupt these processes and lead to health issues.

In the context of a diet, an alkaline diet emphasizes foods that are believed to have an alkalizing effect on the body, helping to maintain a healthy pH balance. These typically include fruits, vegetables, nuts, seeds, and legumes.

How the body maintains its pH balance

Our bodies have a built-in regulatory system to maintain a stable pH level, usually around 7.4 in blood and most other body fluids. This is accomplished through various mechanisms:

- *Buffer Systems*: These are mixtures of the body's own naturally occurring weak acids and their alkaline salts (like bicarbonate ions). They work by neutralizing any excess acid or base that enters the body.
- *Respiration*: Our lungs can also regulate pH by either retaining or releasing carbon dioxide (CO_2), which is acidic. When the body is too acidic, we breathe faster to release more CO_2 and increase the pH. When the body is too alkaline, we breathe slower to retain CO_2 and decrease the pH.
- *Kidneys*: The kidneys further adjust pH by excreting excess acids or bases in urine and reabsorbing bicarbonate from urine.

The role of diet in influencing our body's pH level

The food we eat can influence our body's pH balance. Foods are classified as either acid-forming or alkaline-forming based on the residue they leave in the body after digestion, not whether they are acidic or alkaline themselves. For example, lemons are acidic, but they are alkaline-forming in the body.

Alkaline-forming foods, such as most fruits and vegetables, help maintain a healthy pH balance by neutralizing acid. On the other hand, a diet high in acid-forming foods, like meat, dairy, and processed foods, can lead to a lower (more acidic) pH level in the body. This doesn't mean these foods should be entirely avoided, but they should be balanced with alkaline foods to maintain optimal health.

Remember, while diet can influence your body's pH, it's your body's regulatory systems that maintain the pH within a very narrow, healthy range. An alkaline diet can support these systems but won't drastically alter your body's pH.

How Does Diet Work in Our Body?

When we eat foods, our body breaks them down into smaller molecules that can be absorbed and utilized. These smaller molecules enter the bloodstream and are transported to different parts of the body for various functions. During this process, some foods leave an acidic residue while others leave an alkaline residue in the body.

Once these residues enter the bloodstream, they interact with oxygen and form either acids or bases. Acids are molecules that give up oxygen while bases are molecules that pick up oxygen.

These reactions help maintain our body's pH balance, as the alkaline residues neutralize any excess acid and vice versa. However, if there is an imbalance in our diet, such as consuming too many acid-forming foods, this can cause the body to rely on > its buffering systems to maintain the pH balance. Over time, this can put a strain on these systems and potentially lead to health issues.

So, by consuming an alkaline diet, we are providing our body with more alkaline-forming foods that help maintain a healthy pH balance without relying too much on our body's regulatory systems. This can support optimal health and well-being while also reducing the strain on our body's buffering systems.

Alkaline Aligns with Women for a Specific Purpose

Women can greatly benefit from adopting an alkaline plant-based diet, as it has been shown to improve a variety of health conditions. Here are some specific use cases of how this diet can benefit women with certain diseases:

Osteoporosis

Osteoporosis poses a significant health risk, especially for post-menopausal women. An alkaline plant-based diet is potentially beneficial for those at a higher risk of developing this disease. This diet, abundant in essential nutrients, can aid in strengthening bones and potentially decelerating the progression of osteoporosis.

Moreover, an alkaline diet can enhance bone health by lowering the body's acidity, which often results in calcium loss. Women adhering to such a dietary approach may also reap other health benefits, including enhanced cardiovascular well-being, inflammation reduction, and improved digestion.

Breast Cancer

Breast cancer is a substantial health concern for women worldwide, and dietary habits significantly influence its prevention and management. An alkaline diet might provide some protection against breast cancer. This diet helps maintain a balanced pH in the body, creating an environment less favorable for cancer cell development.

This dietary approach may hinder the growth of these cells. While it doesn't serve as a cure, integrating an alkaline diet could potentially supplement conventional treatment methods, playing a part in a comprehensive strategy for breast cancer prevention.

Polycystic Ovary Syndrome (PCOS)

Polycystic Ovary Syndrome (PCOS) is a prevalent endocrine condition affecting women in their childbearing years. Women with PCOS often struggle with managing their symptoms, which can include weight gain, irregular periods, and acne. An alkaline plant-based diet, low in processed foods and sugars, may provide some relief.

This diet not only aids in weight management but also helps maintain a balanced insulin level, a key concern for women with PCOS. Foods rich in fiber, such as fruits, vegetables, and whole grains, are integral to this diet and can help regulate blood sugar levels, potentially alleviating PCOS symptoms.

Menopause Symptoms

Menopause is a transitional phase in a woman's life marked by hormonal changes leading to symptoms like hot flashes and mood swings. An alkaline plant-based diet could potentially help in easing these symptoms.

This diet, low in processed foods and sugars, can help balance hormones by providing essential nutrients. Moreover, the diet can aid in maintaining a healthy weight, which often becomes a concern during menopause. Thus, adopting such a dietary approach could serve as a natural strategy for managing menopausal symptoms.

Cardiovascular Disease

Cardiovascular disease is a paramount health concern, particularly for women. An alkaline plant-based diet, characterized by its low saturated fat and high fiber content, can be instrumental in managing this risk. This diet aids in lowering cholesterol levels, a key contributor to heart disease. Lower cholesterol reduces the potential for harmful arterial blockages, thereby decreasing the risk of heart-related incidents.

Furthermore, an alkaline diet helps in maintaining optimal pH balance in the body, essential for overall cardiovascular health. It's noteworthy that while diet is crucial, it complements other lifestyle factors like regular physical activity in promoting heart health. The benefits of this diet extend beyond heart disease prevention, contributing positively to general well-being.

Pregnancy Health

Maintaining a healthy pregnancy is crucial, and an alkaline plant-based diet can play a significant role. This diet is rich in essential nutrients that contribute to a healthy pregnancy, like folic acid, iron, and calcium. Folic acid supports neural tube development, iron aids in creating extra blood to supply oxygen to the baby, and calcium strengthens the baby's bones and teeth.

Furthermore, an alkaline diet helps maintain the body's pH balance, which is beneficial for both the mother's and the baby's health. It also assists in reducing pregnancy-related issues such as heartburn and morning sickness. However, it's important to remember that while diet is vital, regular prenatal check-ups and a balanced lifestyle are equally significant during pregnancy.

While an alkaline plant-based diet can complement treatment strategies for these conditions, it should not replace medical treatment. Always consult a healthcare professional before making significant dietary changes.

The Alkaline Plant Based Diet

The Alkaline Plant-Based Diet is a dietary approach that focuses on the consumption of plant-based, alkaline-forming foods like fruits, vegetables, and legumes, while reducing acid-forming foods such as meat, dairy, and processed goods. Its goal is to optimize health by promoting a balanced body pH and nutrient-dense eating.

Principles of Alkaline Plant Based Diet

The Alkaline Plant-Based Diet operates on several key principles:

- *Eat Alkaline Foods*: This diet encourages the consumption of foods that are alkaline-forming in the body, such as fruits, vegetables, nuts, seeds, and legumes.
- *Limit Acidic Foods*: Acid-forming foods like meat, dairy, eggs, grains, and processed foods should be limited or avoided.
- *Whole Foods Focus*: The diet emphasizes eating whole, unprocessed foods for their high nutrient content.

- *Hydration*: Drinking plenty of water, particularly alkaline water, is encouraged to assist in maintaining a balanced pH level in the body.
- *Mindful Eating*: It encourages mindful eating practices, such as chewing thoroughly and eating slowly, to aid digestion and absorption of nutrients.
- *Regular Exercise*: Regular physical activity is also recommended as it can help maintain a healthy pH balance in the body.

Remember, before starting any new diet plan, it's always a good idea to consult with a healthcare professional.

Benefits of Alkaline Plant Based Diet

Incorporating an Alkaline Plant-Based Diet into your lifestyle can bring about a variety of health benefits, including:

- *Balanced Body pH*: By focusing on alkaline-forming foods, it helps maintain a balanced body pH, which is crucial for overall health.
- *Weight Loss*: As the diet focuses on whole, unprocessed foods, it can lead to weight loss due to reduced calorie intake.
- *Improved Digestion*: The high fiber content of plant-based foods can aid digestion and promote gut health.

- *Disease Prevention*: The nutrient-rich foods in this diet can help prevent chronic diseases like heart disease, diabetes, and cancer.
- *Enhanced Energy Levels*: Consuming nutrient-dense, alkaline foods can boost energy levels and overall well-being.
- *Better Skin Health*: The antioxidants in plant-based foods can improve skin health and complexion.

Remember, individual experiences with the diet may vary, and it's essential to consult with a healthcare professional before starting any new diet plan.

Disadvantages of Alkaline Plant Based Diet

While the Alkaline Plant-Based Diet has many benefits, it also comes with a few potential disadvantages:

- *Restrictive*: This diet can be restrictive as it eliminates several food groups, including meat, dairy, and grains, which might make it challenging to follow long-term.
- *Nutrient Deficiencies*: The absence of certain food groups could potentially lead to deficiencies in nutrients like Vitamin B12, iron, calcium, and protein, which are abundant in animal products.
- *Lack of Scientific Evidence*: Some claims about the diet, particularly regarding its ability to change body pH, lack robust scientific backing.

However, the potential benefits of this diet often outweigh these drawbacks. By focusing on nutrient-rich, whole foods, the diet promotes weight loss, improved digestion, disease prevention, enhanced energy levels, and better skin health.

Moreover, potential nutrient deficiencies can be avoided with careful meal planning or appropriate supplementation. So, despite some challenges, many find the Alkaline Plant-Based Diet a worthy approach to promoting overall wellness. It's always best to consult with a healthcare professional before starting any new diet plan.

A 5-Step-by-Step Guide To Getting Started With The Diet

Starting an Alkaline Plant-Based Diet can be a significant lifestyle change, but it doesn't have to be daunting. Here's a simple five-step guide to help you embark on this journey:

Step 1: Educate Yourself

Embarking on the Alkaline Plant-Based Diet journey begins with educating yourself about the fundamentals of this dietary approach. This diet primarily focuses on the consumption of alkaline-forming foods and the reduction, or even elimination, of acid-forming foods.

To get started, it's crucial to understand what makes a food alkaline or acidic. Alkaline foods are those that have a higher pH level, typically above 7, while acidic foods have a lower pH level, usually below 7. The pH level of a food is determined by the residue it leaves in your body after it has been metabolized, not by the pH level of the food itself.

Alkaline-forming foods are predominantly plant-based, including most fruits, vegetables, herbs, nuts, and seeds.

These foods are rich in essential nutrients that promote overall health. They are packed with antioxidants and fiber, which can help flush toxins out of your body, aid in digestion, boost your immune system, and contribute to weight loss.

Acid-forming foods, on the other hand, include meat, dairy, and highly processed foods. These foods are typically high in unhealthy fats, sugars, and artificial additives, which can lead to inflammation, weight gain, and other health problems when consumed in excess.

Your aim in following an Alkaline Plant-Based Diet should be to maximize the intake of alkaline foods and minimize the consumption of acidic ones. However, it's important to remember that balance is key to maintaining good health. Even though the focus is on alkaline foods, it doesn't mean that all acidic foods must be completely omitted. Some acidic foods, like certain whole grains and legumes, still have nutritional value and can be part of a balanced diet.

Educating yourself about the Alkaline Plant-Based Diet is about more than just learning what to eat and what to avoid. It's also about understanding the potential benefits and challenges of this diet, how it can impact your overall health, and how to make it work for your specific needs and lifestyle. This knowledge will empower you to make informed decisions about your diet and help you successfully transition to a healthier way of eating.

Step 2: Purge Your Pantry

The second step in transitioning to the Alkaline Plant-Based Diet involves a thorough purge of your pantry and refrigerator. This step is crucial as it removes temptation and sets up your environment for success, making it easier for you to stick to your new eating habits.

Start by identifying all the acid-forming foods in your kitchen. These are typically meat products, dairy items, and heavily processed foods. Acid-forming foods also include certain grains, legumes, and most beverages aside from water. Don't forget to check your condiments, sauces, and dressings, which often contain hidden sugars and unhealthy fats, making them highly acidic.

Once you've identified these foods, it's time to remove them. You can donate unopened non-perishable items to a local food bank or share them with friends or family who aren't following an alkaline diet. For perishable items, plan meals around them until they're used up, to avoid wastage.

Having a clean slate doesn't mean your pantry and refrigerator should be empty. Replace the removed items with alkaline-forming foods. Stock up on a variety of fresh fruits and vegetables, both for cooking and snacking. Fill your pantry with nuts and seeds for protein, and whole grains and legumes for fiber. You should also consider investing in some healthy oils like olive oil or avocado oil for cooking.

Don't forget to also consider your drinks. Sugary sodas and alcohol are highly acidic. Instead, opt for alkaline water, herbal teas, or natural fruit juices. Hydration is key in any diet, and more so in an alkaline one.

By purging your pantry and filling it back up with healthier alternatives, you're not only making a physical transformation in your kitchen but also taking a significant psychological step towards embracing your new lifestyle. This clear commitment will set the stage for your successful transition to the Alkaline Plant-Based Diet.

Step 3: Meal Planning

Now that your pantry and refrigerator are stocked with alkaline-forming foods, it's time to plan your meals. Meal planning is a crucial step in maintaining a healthy diet, as it allows you to ensure you're getting a balanced intake of nutrients each day.

Firstly, it's important to remember that variety is key to a healthy diet. Aim to include a wide range of fruits, vegetables, legumes, nuts, and seeds in your meals throughout the week. Different foods offer different nutrients, so eating a diverse range of foods will help ensure you're getting all the vitamins, minerals, and other nutrients your body needs to function optimally.

When planning your meals, consider the balance of macronutrients—carbohydrates, proteins, and fats. Despite being a plant-based diet, an alkaline diet can still provide all the necessary nutrients your body needs.

Carbohydrates can come from fruits, vegetables, and whole grains. These foods are not only alkaline-forming but also high in fiber, which aids digestion and keeps you feeling full longer.

Proteins are essential for building and repairing body tissue, among other functions. In an alkaline diet, good sources of protein include legumes like lentils and chickpeas, and nuts and seeds like almonds and chia seeds.

Healthy fats are also vital for your body's functioning, including supporting cell growth and protecting your organs. Avocados, olives, and seeds like flax seeds and chia seeds are excellent sources of healthy fats in an alkaline diet.

As you plan your meals, remember to pay attention to portion sizes. Even healthy foods can lead to weight gain if consumed in excess. Use measuring cups or a food scale to ensure you're eating appropriate portions.

Finally, be sure to plan for snacks as well. Keeping healthy, alkaline-forming snacks on hand can help you avoid reaching for acidic, processed foods when hunger strikes between meals. Consider options like fresh fruits, raw nuts, or hummus with vegetable sticks.

Incorporating meal planning into your routine not only helps you stay on track with your Alkaline Plant-Based Diet but also reduces stress and saves time in the long run. By knowing what you'll eat in advance, you can avoid last-minute unhealthy food choices and enjoy a diverse, balanced, and nutrient-rich diet.

Step 4: Hydrate Well

Hydration plays a pivotal role in the Alkaline Plant-Based Diet, as well as in overall health. Water is essential for nearly every bodily function, from regulating body temperature to flushing out toxins and aiding digestion.

In an Alkaline Plant-Based Diet, the goal should be to drink at least eight glasses of water every day. This is a general guideline, but individual needs may vary based on factors like age, sex, weight, physical activity levels, and climate. For instance, if you're physically active or live in a hot climate, you might need more than eight glasses.

The type of water you drink can also impact your body's pH balance. If possible, consider incorporating alkaline water into your routine. Alkaline water typically has a pH level of 8 or 9, higher than regular drinking water, which generally has a neutral pH of 7. Some studies suggest that drinking alkaline water can help neutralize acid in the body, boost metabolism, and improve the absorption of nutrients. However, more research is needed to fully understand its potential benefits and risks.

In addition to drinking water, you can also hydrate by consuming foods with high water content. Many fruits and vegetables, such as cucumbers, watermelon, oranges, and strawberries, are composed of over 90% water. These foods not only contribute to your hydration goals but also provide a variety of vitamins, minerals, and antioxidants that promote health.

Remember, while hydration is crucial, it's equally important not to overdo it. Drinking too much water can lead to water intoxication, a serious condition that can disrupt your body's electrolyte balance. As always, balance is key. Listen to your body's thirst cues and adjust your fluid intake accordingly.

By prioritizing hydration, you're not just supporting your transition to the Alkaline Plant-Based Diet but also promoting optimal health and well-being.

Step 5: Track Your Progress

Embarking on a new diet is a journey, and like any journey, it's important to track your progress. As you transition to the Alkaline Plant-Based Diet, pay close attention to how you're feeling both physically and mentally.

Take note of any changes in your energy levels, digestion, skin condition, weight, and overall well-being. This will help you gauge how well your body is responding to the dietary changes. Keep a food diary if needed, recording what you eat and how you feel afterward. This can be an effective tool for identifying foods that make you feel good and those that don't sit well with you.

However, if you notice negative symptoms such as constant fatigue, weakness, dizziness, or other health concerns, it's crucial not to ignore these signs. Don't hesitate to consult with a healthcare professional or a registered dietitian. They can provide guidance and help you adjust your diet to ensure you're getting all the nutrients you need. It's essential to remember that while the Alkaline Plant-Based Diet has many benefits, it should not compromise your overall health.

Change indeed takes time and requires patience. Transitioning to a new way of eating won't happen overnight, and it's okay to have some bumps along the way. Be kind to yourself during this process. Celebrate each step forward, no matter how small it may seem. Every healthy choice you make brings you closer to fully embracing your new Alkaline Plant-Based Diet.

In due course, with consistency and balance, you'll start to see the positive impacts of this lifestyle change. You may experience improved digestion, clearer skin, increased energy levels, and better overall health. These benefits will serve as motivation to continue on your journey toward a healthier, more balanced lifestyle. Remember, the goal isn't perfection but progress, and every step forward is a victory worth celebrating.

Foods to Eat and to Avoid

In an Alkaline Plant-Based Diet, the goal is to consume foods that help maintain a slightly alkaline pH level in your body. Here's a list of foods to eat and avoid:

Foods to Eat

The alkaline diet primarily consists of whole foods with a high pH level, which are believed to help in balancing your body's acidity levels. Here's a detailed list of some common alkaline foods:

- ***Fruits***: Apples, cherries, pineapples, and other fruits are excellent sources of alkaline. Fruits are packed with antioxidants and fiber, which aid digestion and boost immune health.
- ***Vegetables***: Non-starchy vegetables like beets, broccoli, mushrooms, peas, and tomatoes along with leafy greens such as spinach, kale, and arugula are highly alkaline. These are rich in vitamins, minerals, and fiber, promoting heart health and aiding digestion.
- ***Beans/Legumes/Roots***: Lentils and roots like lotus root or burdock are alkaline-forming foods. They provide a good source of plant-based protein and fiber, helping to maintain stable blood sugar levels.

- ***Nuts and Seeds***: Almonds are particularly alkaline. Other nuts and seeds also contribute to alkalinity. These are rich in healthy fats, fiber, and protein, promoting satiety and heart health.
- ***Drinks***: Unsweetened fruit juices, almond milk, and mineral soda water are alkaline beverages. These hydrating options can help flush toxins from the body and aid in digestion.

Tips on Incorporating These Foods into Daily Meals

1. Start your day with a piece of fruit or a green smoothie.
2. Add a variety of vegetables to your meals, either as a salad, a side dish, or incorporated into main dishes.
3. Include a serving of beans or lentils in your meals for added protein and fiber.
4. Snack on a handful of almonds or add them to your salads and dishes for a crunchy texture.
5. Replace sugary drinks with unsweetened fruit juices or mineral soda water.

Remember, while the alkaline diet can be healthy due to its emphasis on fruits and vegetables, it's not necessary to strictly follow this eating pattern. A balanced diet that includes a variety of foods from all food groups is the key to good health.

Foods to Avoid

Certain foods can contribute to acidity in the body. Here's a list of some common ones that you might want to avoid or limit on the alkaline diet:

- *Alcohol*: All types of alcohol are acidic.
- *Cheese*: Most cheeses are acidic, especially processed cheese.
- *Eggs*: Eggs are considered moderately acidic.
- *Fish*: Most types of fish are acidic.
- *Grains*: Many grains, including wheat and oats, are acidic.
- *Meat*: Red meats are highly acidic.
- *Milk*: Cow's milk and most dairy products are acidic.
- *Processed Foods*: These often contain preservatives and artificial ingredients that can make them highly acidic.
- *Soda*: Carbonated drinks, especially those with sugar, are very acidic.

Explanation of Why These Foods Are Not Ideal for the Alkaline Diet

The alkaline diet is based on the idea that consuming too many acid-forming foods can cause an imbalance in your body's pH levels, potentially leading to various health issues. The foods listed above are considered acidic, meaning they may lower the pH of your body fluids. Over time, this could lead to a condition known as acidosis, which can cause symptoms like fatigue, shortness of breath, and confusion.

Tips on Finding Healthier Alternatives to These Foods

- *Alcohol*: Opt for non-alcoholic beverages, such as herbal teas or infused water.
- *Cheese*: Try plant-based cheeses made from nuts or soy.
- *Eggs*: Substitute eggs with flaxseeds or chia seeds in recipes.
- *Fish*: Swap out fish with plant-based proteins like lentils or tofu.
- *Grains*: Choose alkaline grains like amaranth, quinoa, and millet.
- *Meat*: Replace meat with plant-based proteins such as beans, lentils, and tempeh.
- *Milk*: Opt for alkaline alternatives like almond milk or coconut milk.
- *Processed Foods*: Make homemade versions of your favorite foods to avoid preservatives and artificial ingredients.
- *Soda*: Swap soda for mineral water, herbal teas, or homemade fruit juices.

Remember, it's not necessary to completely eliminate these foods from your diet. The key is balance and moderation. Always consult with a healthcare professional before making significant changes to your diet.

Week 1: Heating It Up

Now that you know what you can get from the alkaline diet, it is important to know whether it is the right diet for you. Ask the following questions to yourself:

- Do I want to have a healthy, fit, and toned body?
- Am I willing to accept the challenge of eating only fruits and vegetables?
- Do I want to achieve my goals towards a healthier lifestyle?

If you answered all three questions without hesitation, then you have passed the first phase!

Assessing yourself whether you can do the diet or not is a way to mentally prepare for what will come about when you are already doing the diet. It involves managing your expectations and what steps you are likely to take once you are in the middle of the diet.

Since it is a lifestyle change that requires tons of discipline and willpower, most people steer away from deciding to switch diets, even though it will benefit them in the long run.

It is good to know though that you are eager to cross the bridge towards a healthier lifestyle. At this phase, it is something to be proud of already!

Assessing also involves instilling your goals in mind and making them a driving force for you to continue. Your goal may vary from weight loss, wanting to have healthier habits, reducing your vulnerability to certain diseases, or maybe all of them. Who knows, right? Whatever they may be, these are what should be etched in your mind from the start until the end.

After assessing, you can now start to plan how you will execute the diet. Listed below are some guide questions that can help you properly plan how you will start the alkaline plant-based diet:

- How often do I need to go to the grocery store to buy the products I need?
- What meals do I need to eat?
- Do I need to learn how to cook dishes?
- Do not be overwhelmed because this guide will help you answer the questions above!
- How often do I need to go to the grocery store to buy the products I need?

The frequency of your grocery shopping depends on you! It may be weekly, monthly, or even twice a week. However, since the food you are recommended to eat is better when it's freshly picked, you can consider shopping weekly. Fruits and vegetables rot easily, especially in humid weather. If you have a refrigerator, then that would not be a problem.

But buying in small bunches is recommended if you are going to use the ingredients sparingly. So, planning your meals will help you with what you need to buy when grocery shopping. This leads us to the next question...

What meals do I need to eat?

Fruits and vegetables have a wide array of flavors and aromas themselves. Some can be eaten raw, blanched, fried, grilled, or even tossed in a salad— the possibilities are endless. Depending on your preference for dishes, you can choose to cook them or eat them raw.

This diet might even make you a cook since you can experiment with different flavors of different dishes that you can create with your fruits and vegetables. And down to the next question...

Do I need to learn how to cook dishes?

No. You do not need to learn how to cook. But, it is highly recommended. If you are a busy person who eats out more, the alkaline plant-based diet will still be achievable. However, you should be careful in choosing what food you are ordering by scanning and asking the servers what ingredients they use in your food. Because some might contain more acidic foods. And you do not want that in your diet.

Cooking, however, will help you become more confident with the food you eat without worrying about ingesting acidic food. Moreover, you can prepare your dishes ahead of time so all you need to do is take them out of the refrigerator and reheat them. This also puts you in control of what you want to eat for the day or the week.

Now that you have laid out a plan to execute your starting point, commitment is the only thing that will seal the deal.

Week 2: Starting the Engine

Since you have already planned your alkaline scheme, it is time to bring your all in! Put your plans into action by making a meal plan, preparing your grocery list and grocery schedule, and learning how to cook (if you are a newbie cook)!

It can be nerve-wracking to go to the grocery store especially when you just started changing your diet. You may see your old acidic favorites and put them in your cart as an instinct, but you need to get rid of those habits.

So, below are some tips on how to face the grocery battlefield:

Make a list

Listing is still the best way to track what you should buy. You may categorize them into needs or wants, or what to buy in bulk or little amounts. This is also where you will put the things you need to buy based on the meal plan that you created.

Stick to the list

Although it is tempting to buy hotdogs or a tub of ice cream, remember the reason why you started this diet. Parting is always a sweet sorrow, and to promise you, the results of the alkaline plant-based diet are sweeter. Sticking to the list also makes it easier since it will make you have shorter trips to the grocery store. Instead of ogling to other grocery aisles, you will go directly to where you need to go.

Check which products are in season

Some fruits and vegetables are available all year round, and some are only harvested when they are in season. But it is important to note that even if they are available all year, these products still have a particular season where the harvest is much more delicious and plentiful!

For example, spinach is available throughout the year. They can be bought fresh or frozen. But they are in their best shape between March and June. So, you may want to indulge yourself with spinach during those months.

The products that you bought from the groceries are all aligned with your meal plan. So, making your meal plan would help you a lot in doing other things such as grocery shopping.

How do you make a meal plan?

Know your preferences

You already know that alkaline foods should be the only thing that you will eat from now on. So, knowing what you can eat within this food bracket is important. Incorporating your food preferences into your meal plan would also make you look forward to your future meals, as you can put all your favorites in a week's meal. Everything will solely depend on you.

Incorporate moderation, variety, and balance

In making your meal plan, it is important to incorporate these nutrition principles to make meals more achievable and palatable. Moderation refers to controlling the amount of food you eat. Even though it is all fruits and vegetables in the alkaline plant-based diet, it does not mean that you can eat ten plates of these.

Counting calories will be helpful to know the amount of food you should eat per meal. This is also helpful if you want to lose weight! Just lessen the calories and see the results! Next, variety is also important so that you will not get tired of eating the same textures every time. You can have something crunchy, and then soft, and creamy in a single meal.

This will make your dish palatable and pleasing to your tongue as well. Lastly, balancing your meals is important for you to get the recommended intake of food and nutrients.

Balancing your meals ensures that you are getting the optimum nutrients for the day. You can check MyPlate to help you in planning the portions of food on your plate. Make sure to replace acidic animal protein with vegetable or fruit protein!

Learn basic cooking techniques

Since you are preparing your meal plan, anyway, might as well cook them on your own! Fruits and vegetables are easy ingredients to cook. You can cook them raw, boil them, simmer, heat, fry, grill, anything... You can even put them into hot water, and they are ready to eat. Unlike acidic products, vegetables and fruits can be cooked for under 10 minutes or less, depending on their structure. If you are lazy, you can slice fruits and you already have your breakfast!

Now that you have everything you need to have and all the things you need to learn, you are ready to start the diet! To help you begin this journey, a weekly meal plan is specially crafted for you! The meal plan consists of dishes and snacks that you can try to have a head start in that lifestyle change. Some recipes are also available so you can visualize how you will prepare for your first week of the alkaline diet.

7-Day Sample Meal Plan

This chapter provides a sample meal plan to help you start your alkaline diet. This will give you an idea of how to structure your meals and also provide some inspiration for dishes that fit into the alkaline diet.

Sunday

Breakfast: Quinoa porridge with almond milk, topped with sliced banana and a sprinkle of chia seeds

Lunch: Chickpea salad with spinach, cucumber, bell peppers, and a lemon-tahini dressing

Dinner: Stuffed bell peppers with quinoa, black beans, corn, and avocado

Snack: Handful of almonds

Monday

Breakfast: Green smoothie made with spinach, banana, and a spoonful of almond butter

Lunch: Lentil soup with a side of mixed greens

Dinner: Baked sweet potato topped with black beans, corn, and avocado

Snack: Freshly cut watermelon cubes

Tuesday

Breakfast: Chia seed pudding with almond milk, sweetened with a touch of maple syrup and topped with fresh berries

Lunch: Quinoa salad with roasted vegetables and a drizzle of olive oil

Dinner: Grilled zucchini and eggplant skewers with a side of millet.

Snack: A handful of sunflower seeds

Wednesday

Breakfast: Avocado toast on sprouted grain bread with a sprinkle of hemp seeds

Lunch: Vegetable stir-fry with tofu served over brown rice

Dinner: Lentil and vegetable curry served with quinoa

Snack: Freshly cut pineapple chunks

Thursday

Breakfast: Smoothie bowl with blended frozen berries, banana, and almond milk, topped with granola and coconut flakes

Lunch: Chickpea and vegetable wrap with whole grain tortilla

Dinner: Spaghetti squash with homemade tomato sauce and a sprinkle of nutritional yeast

Snack: A handful of pumpkin seeds

Friday

Breakfast: Overnight oats with almond milk, topped with sliced peaches and a sprinkle of flaxseeds

Lunch: Baked falafel salad with cucumber, tomato, and a drizzle of tahini dressing

Dinner: Stuffed portobello mushrooms with quinoa and spinach

Snack: Freshly cut cantaloupe

Saturday

Breakfast: Green juice made with cucumber, spinach, apple, and lemon

Lunch: Lentil and vegetable stuffed bell peppers

Dinner: Vegan chili made with kidney beans, black beans, corn, and a variety of vegetables

Snack: A bowl of mixed berries

Remember, the key to a successful diet plan is to adjust it according to your taste and nutritional needs. Enjoy exploring these meal ideas and feel free to make them your own!

Curated Recipes

These recipes are carefully selected to provide a diverse and balanced range of nutrients for a healthy and sustainable plant-based diet. Whether you are new to the world of veganism or looking for some fresh meal ideas, these curated recipes will surely inspire and satisfy your taste buds.

Quinoa Porridge

Ingredients:

- 1/2 cup of quinoa
- 2 cups of unsweetened almond milk
- 1 ripe banana (sliced)
- 1 tablespoon chia seeds
- Optional: natural sweetener like agave nectar or pure maple syrup to taste

Instructions:

1. Rinse the quinoa under cold water until the water runs clear. This is an important step to remove the natural coating of quinoa that can make it taste bitter.
2. In a medium-sized pot, combine the rinsed quinoa and almond milk. Bring the mixture to a boil over medium-high heat.
3. Once it reaches a boil, reduce the heat to low, cover the pot, and let it simmer. Cook the quinoa for about 15 minutes, or until it becomes soft and the liquid has been absorbed.
4. While the quinoa is cooking, slice your banana into thin discs.
5. Once the quinoa is cooked, remove it from heat and let it sit for 5 minutes with the lid on.
6. Fluff the cooked quinoa with a fork, then divide it into bowls.

7. Top each bowl with sliced bananas, a sprinkle of chia seeds, and if desired, a drizzle of your chosen sweetener.
8. Serve warm and enjoy!

Chickpea Salad with Lemon-Tahini Dressing

Ingredients:

For the salad:

- 1 can of chickpeas, rinsed and drained
- 2 cups of fresh spinach leaves
- 1 cucumber, diced
- 1 bell pepper, diced

For the dressing:

- 2 tablespoons of tahini
- Juice of 1 lemon
- 2 tablespoons of water
- Salt to taste

Instructions:

1. Begin by preparing your vegetables. Rinse the spinach leaves thoroughly, dice the cucumber and bell pepper into bite-sized pieces.
2. In a large bowl, combine the rinsed and drained chickpeas, spinach leaves, diced cucumber, and bell pepper.
3. Now, let's prepare the dressing. In a small bowl, combine the tahini and lemon juice. Stir until well mixed.
4. Add water to the tahini-lemon mixture, one tablespoon at a time, stirring after each addition. Keep adding

water until you achieve your desired dressing consistency.
5. Season the dressing with salt, to taste.
6. Pour the dressing over the salad ingredients in a large bowl.
7. Toss the salad until all the ingredients are evenly coated with the dressing.
8. Serve immediately, or refrigerate for later use.

Stuffed Bell Peppers

Ingredients:

- 4 bell peppers
- 1 cup cooked quinoa
- 1 can black beans, rinsed and drained
- 1 cup corn (fresh, canned, or frozen)
- 1 ripe avocado, diced
- Salt and pepper to taste

For the garnish:

- Fresh cilantro leaves
- Lime wedges

Instructions:

1. Preheat your oven to 375°F (190°C).
2. Cut off the tops of the bell peppers and remove the seeds inside. Set these aside.
3. In a large bowl, combine the cooked quinoa, rinsed black beans, corn, and diced avocado. Mix well.
4. Season the mixture with salt and pepper, to taste.
5. Spoon this mixture into each bell pepper until they are filled to the top.
6. Place the stuffed peppers in a baking dish and bake for about 20-25 minutes, or until the peppers are tender.

7. Once done, remove from the oven and allow to cool slightly.
8. Garnish with fresh cilantro leaves and serve with lime wedges on the side.

Green Smoothie

Ingredients:

- 2 cups of fresh spinach
- 1 ripe banana
- 1 tablespoon of almond butter
- 1 cup of almond milk or water
- Optional: Ice cubes

Instructions:

1. Rinse the fresh spinach under cold water.
2. Peel and slice the ripe banana.
3. In a blender, add the rinsed spinach, sliced banana, almond butter, and almond milk or water.
4. Blend until the mixture is smooth and creamy. If you prefer your smoothies to be cold, you can add some ice cubes and blend again until smooth.
5. Pour the smoothie into a glass and enjoy immediately!

Lentil Soup with a Side of Mixed Greens

Ingredients:

For the soup:

- 1 cup dried lentils, rinsed
- 4 cups water or vegetable broth
- 1 onion, diced
- 2 cloves garlic, minced
- 1 carrot, diced
- 1 celery stalk, diced
- Salt and pepper to taste

For the mixed greens:

- 4 cups mixed greens (spinach, kale, arugula, etc.)
- 1 tablespoon olive oil
- Juice of half a lemon
- Salt and pepper to taste

Instructions:

1. In a large pot, add the lentils, water or broth, onion, garlic, carrot, and celery.
2. Bring the mixture to a boil over medium-high heat.
3. Once boiling, reduce the heat to low and let the soup simmer for about 30 minutes, or until the lentils are tender.
4. Season the soup with salt and pepper, to taste.

5. While the soup is simmering, prepare the mixed greens. In a large bowl, add the mixed greens, olive oil, and lemon juice.
6. Toss the greens until they are evenly coated with the oil and lemon juice. Season with salt and pepper, to taste.
7. Serve the lentil soup hot with the mixed greens on the side.

Baked Sweet Potato

Ingredients:

- 2 large sweet potatoes
- 1 can black beans, rinsed and drained
- 1 cup corn (fresh, canned, or frozen)
- 1 ripe avocado, diced
- Salt and pepper to taste

For the garnish:

- Fresh cilantro leaves
- Lime wedges

Instructions:

1. Preheat your oven to 400°F (200°C).
2. Wash the sweet potatoes and prick them several times with a fork.
3. Place the sweet potatoes on a baking sheet and bake for about 45 minutes, or until they are tender.
4. While the sweet potatoes are baking, prepare the toppings. In a bowl, combine the rinsed black beans, corn, and diced avocado. Mix well.
5. Season the mixture with salt and pepper, to taste.
6. Once the sweet potatoes are done, remove them from the oven and let them cool slightly.
7. Cut a slit on the top of each sweet potato and push the ends towards the center to open.

8. Spoon the black bean, corn, and avocado mixture onto each sweet potato.
9. Garnish with fresh cilantro leaves and serve with lime wedges on the side.

Chia Seed Pudding with Almond Milk

Ingredients:

- 1/4 cup chia seeds
- 1 cup almond milk
- 1-2 tablespoons maple syrup (adjust to taste)
- 1/2 cup fresh berries (raspberries, blueberries, strawberries, etc.)

Instructions:

1. In a bowl or mason jar, combine the chia seeds and almond milk.
2. Stir well to ensure all the chia seeds are immersed in the milk.
3. Sweeten the mixture with maple syrup, adjusting the amount to your liking.
4. Cover the bowl or jar and refrigerate for at least 2 hours, or overnight. The chia seeds will absorb the almond milk and expand, creating a pudding-like consistency.
5. Before serving, give the pudding a good stir to break up any clumps.
6. Top the pudding with fresh berries.
7. Enjoy immediately, or store in the refrigerator for up to three days.

Quinoa Salad with Roasted Vegetables

Ingredients:

- 1 cup quinoa
- 2 cups water
- 2 cups assorted vegetables (such as bell peppers, zucchini, eggplant, etc.), chopped
- 2 tablespoons olive oil, divided
- Salt and pepper to taste
- A handful of fresh herbs (like parsley or basil), chopped

Instructions:

1. Preheat your oven to 400°F (200°C).
2. In a saucepan, bring the water to a boil. Add the quinoa, reduce the heat to low, cover, and simmer for about 15 minutes, or until all the water is absorbed.
3. While the quinoa is cooking, prepare the vegetables. Toss the chopped vegetables with 1 tablespoon of olive oil and season with salt and pepper.
4. Spread the vegetables out on a baking sheet in a single layer. Roast in the preheated oven for about 20 minutes, or until they are tender and slightly browned.
5. Once the quinoa is done, fluff it with a fork and transfer it to a large bowl.
6. Add the roasted vegetables to the quinoa and mix well.

7. Drizzle the remaining 1 tablespoon of olive oil over the salad and toss to combine.
8. Sprinkle the fresh herbs on top of the salad before serving.

Grilled Zucchini and Eggplant Skewers

Ingredients:

- 1 large zucchini
- 1 large eggplant
- 2 tablespoons olive oil
- Salt and pepper to taste
- 1 cup millet
- 2 cups water

Instructions:

1. Preheat your grill or grill pan to medium-high heat.
2. Cut the zucchini and eggplant into 1-inch chunks.
3. Thread the chunks onto skewers, alternating between zucchini and eggplant.
4. Brush the skewers with olive oil and season with salt and pepper.
5. Grill the skewers for about 10 minutes, turning occasionally, until the vegetables are tender and have grill marks.
6. While the skewers are grilling, prepare the millet. In a saucepan, bring the water to a boil.
7. Add the millet, reduce the heat to low, cover, and simmer for about 20 minutes, or until all the water is absorbed.

8. Use a fork to gently separate the grains of the cooked millet.
9. Serve the grilled skewers with a side of millet.

Vegetable Stir-Fry with Tofu

Ingredients:

- 1 cup brown rice
- 2 cups water
- 1 block firm tofu
- 3 tablespoons olive oil, divided
- 2 cups assorted vegetables (such as bell peppers, broccoli, carrots, etc.), chopped
- 2 cloves garlic, minced
- 1 tablespoon soy sauce or tamari
- Salt and pepper to taste

Instructions:

1. In a saucepan, bring the water to a boil. Add the brown rice, reduce the heat to low, cover, and let it simmer for about 45 minutes, or until all the water is absorbed.
2. While the rice is cooking, prepare the tofu. Drain and press the tofu to remove excess moisture, then cut it into cubes.
3. Heat 2 tablespoons of olive oil in a large skillet or wok over medium-high heat. Add the tofu cubes and cook until they are golden brown on all sides. Remove the tofu from the skillet and set aside.
4. In the same skillet, add the remaining 1 tablespoon of olive oil. Add the garlic and cook for about 30 seconds, until fragrant.

5. Add the chopped vegetables to the skillet. Stir-fry for about 5-7 minutes until the vegetables are tender-crisp.
6. Return the tofu to the skillet. Add the soy sauce or tamari, and season with salt and pepper. Stir well to combine.
7. Once the brown rice is done, fluff it with a fork.
8. Serve the vegetable stir-fry over the brown rice.

Lentil and Vegetable Curry served with Quinoa

Ingredients:

- 1 cup quinoa
- 2 cups water
- 1 cup lentils
- 3 cups vegetable broth
- 2 tablespoons olive oil
- 1 onion, chopped
- 2 cloves garlic, minced
- 1 tablespoon curry powder
- 2 cups assorted vegetables (such as bell peppers, carrots, zucchini, etc.), chopped
- Salt and pepper to taste

Instructions:

1. In a saucepan, bring the water to a boil. Add the quinoa, reduce the heat to low, cover, and simmer for about 15 minutes, or until all the water is absorbed.
2. In another saucepan, add the lentils and vegetable broth. Bring to a boil, then reduce the heat to low, cover, and simmer for about 20 minutes, or until the lentils are tender.
3. While the quinoa and lentils are cooking, heat the olive oil in a large skillet over medium heat. Add the onion and garlic and cook until the onion is translucent.

4. Add the curry powder to the skillet and stir well to combine. Cook for a minute until fragrant.
5. Add the chopped vegetables to the skillet and cook for about 5-7 minutes, until they're tender.
6. Once the lentils are done, drain any excess broth and add them to the skillet. Mix well to combine.
7. Season the curry with salt and pepper to taste.
8. Serve the lentil and vegetable curry over the cooked quinoa.

Spaghetti Squash with Homemade Tomato Sauce

Ingredients:

- 1 spaghetti squash
- 2 tablespoons olive oil
- Salt and pepper to taste
- 4 ripe tomatoes, chopped
- 2 cloves garlic, minced
- 1 onion, chopped
- 1 tablespoon dried basil
- 1 tablespoon dried oregano
- 2 tablespoons nutritional yeast

Instructions:

1. Preheat your oven to 400°F (200°C). Cut the spaghetti squash in half lengthwise and scoop out the seeds.
2. Brush the inside of each half with olive oil and season with salt and pepper. Place the halves cut side down on a baking sheet.
3. Roast in the oven for about 40 minutes, or until the flesh is tender and can be easily scraped out with a fork.
4. While the squash is roasting, prepare the tomato sauce. In a large skillet, heat the remaining olive oil over medium heat.

5. Add the onion and garlic to the skillet and cook until the onion is translucent.
6. Add the chopped tomatoes, basil, and oregano to the skillet. Simmer for about 20 minutes, or until the sauce has thickened.
7. Once the spaghetti squash is done, let it cool for a few minutes before using a fork to scrape out the spaghetti-like strands.
8. Serve the spaghetti squash topped with the homemade tomato sauce and a sprinkle of nutritional yeast.

Baked Falafel Salad

Ingredients:

For the falafel:

- 1 cup dried chickpeas, soaked overnight
- 1/2 large onion, roughly chopped
- 2 tablespoons fresh parsley, chopped
- 2 tablespoons fresh cilantro, chopped
- 1 teaspoon lemon juice
- 1 teaspoon olive oil
- 1 teaspoon cumin
- Salt and black pepper to taste

For the salad:

- 2 cups mixed greens
- 1 cucumber, diced
- 1 tomato, diced

For the tahini dressing:

- 1/4 cup tahini
- 2 tablespoons lemon juice
- 1 tablespoon olive oil
- Salt and black pepper to taste

Instructions:

1. Preheat your oven to 375°F (190°C).

2. Drain the chickpeas and place them in a food processor along with the onion, parsley, cilantro, lemon juice, olive oil, cumin, salt, and pepper. Process until smooth.
3. Shape the mixture into small patties and place them on a baking sheet lined with parchment paper.
4. Bake for about 25-30 minutes, or until the falafels are golden brown and crispy.
5. While the falafels are baking, prepare the salad by combining the mixed greens, cucumber, and tomato in a large bowl.
6. For the tahini dressing, whisk together the tahini, lemon juice, olive oil, salt, and pepper in a small bowl.
7. Once the falafels are done, let them cool for a few minutes before adding them to the salad.
8. Drizzle the salad with the tahini dressing.

Stuffed Portobello Mushrooms with Quinoa and Spinach

Ingredients:

- 4 large portobello mushrooms
- 1 cup quinoa
- 2 cups vegetable broth or water
- 2 tablespoons olive oil
- 1 onion, chopped
- 2 cloves garlic, minced
- 2 cups fresh spinach
- Salt and pepper to taste
- 2 tablespoons nutritional yeast (optional)

Instructions:

1. Preheat your oven to 375°F (190°C). Remove the stems from the portobello mushrooms and set the caps aside.
2. Rinse the quinoa under cold water until the water runs clear.
3. In a saucepan, bring the vegetable broth or water to a boil. Add the quinoa, reduce heat to low, cover, and let simmer for about 15 minutes, or until all the liquid is absorbed.
4. While the quinoa is cooking, heat the olive oil in a skillet over medium heat. Add the onion and garlic, and sauté until the onion is translucent.

5. Add the spinach to the skillet and cook until it's wilted. Season with salt and pepper.
6. Once the quinoa is done, add it to the skillet and stir to combine with the spinach mixture.
7. Spoon the quinoa and spinach mixture into the mushroom caps and sprinkle with nutritional yeast if using.
8. Place the stuffed mushrooms on a baking sheet and bake for about 20 minutes, or until the mushrooms are tender.

Vegan Chili

Ingredients:

- 1 tablespoon olive oil
- 1 onion, chopped
- 2 cloves garlic, minced
- 1 bell pepper, chopped
- 1 zucchini, chopped
- 1 carrot, chopped
- 1 cup corn kernels (fresh, frozen, or canned)
- 1 can (15 oz) kidney beans, drained and rinsed
- 1 can (15 oz) black beans, drained and rinsed
- 1 can (28 oz) crushed tomatoes
- 2 tablespoons chili powder
- 1 teaspoon ground cumin
- Salt and pepper to taste

Instructions:

1. Heat the olive oil in a large pot over medium heat. Add the onion and garlic and sauté until the onion is translucent.
2. Add the bell pepper, zucchini, and carrot to the pot. Cook, stirring occasionally, for about 5 minutes, or until the vegetables are tender.
3. Add the corn, kidney beans, black beans, and crushed tomatoes to the pot. Stir to combine.

4. Add chili powder, cumin, salt, and pepper to the mixture for flavor. Mix once more to ensure the spices are spread uniformly through the mixture.
5. Lower the heat to a minimum, secure the lid on the pot, and allow the chili to gently cook for roughly 30 minutes so the various tastes can blend harmoniously.
6. Taste and adjust seasonings if necessary.

Green Juice made with Cucumber, Spinach, Apple, and Lemon

Ingredients:

- 1 large cucumber
- 2 cups fresh spinach
- 1 green apple
- 1 lemon

Instructions:

1. Wash all the fruits and vegetables thoroughly.
2. Cut the cucumber and apple into pieces that are small enough to fit into your juicer's feed tube.
3. If you have an organic lemon, you can juice it with the peel-on for extra nutrients. If it's not organic, it's best to remove the peel to avoid any pesticides.
4. Start your juicer and feed the cucumber, spinach, apple, and lemon through it.
5. Pour the juice into a glass and stir well.
6. It's best to drink your green juice immediately to get the most nutrients, but you can also store it in an airtight container in the fridge for up to 24 hours.

Conclusion

Congratulations on reaching the end of this comprehensive guide to an alkaline plant-based diet. You've taken in a wealth of information, and we're proud of the steps you're taking to revolutionize your health and lifestyle.

Your journey towards adopting an alkaline plant-based diet is an admirable one, steeped in dedication, conscious decision-making, and a deep desire for optimal health. The fact that you've made it this far shows your commitment to understanding the ins and outs of this diet, and for that, we applaud you.

Understanding the alkaline plant-based diet is not just about recognizing the types of foods you should eat. It's also about comprehending how these foods interact with your body, fostering an internal environment that encourages health and discourages disease. By choosing to consume primarily alkaline-forming foods while minimizing acid-forming ones, you're setting yourself up for a life of improved wellness.

As you move forward, remember that this is not merely a diet—it's a lifestyle change. You're choosing to nourish your body with the best nature has to offer, and in return, you'll experience benefits like increased energy, improved digestion, better sleep, weight loss, and so much more.

Remember, it's okay to have questions or face challenges along the way. It's all part of the process. Don't be discouraged if you stumble or find it difficult to fully embrace this lifestyle at first. Be patient with yourself. You're making significant changes, and it's natural to need time to adjust.

Be proud of each step you take, no matter how small. Every alkaline, plant-based meal you consume is a victory. Each time you resist the temptation of acid-forming foods, you're proving to yourself just how strong and committed you are.

In essence, an alkaline plant-based diet is about more than what's on your plate—it's about embracing a healthier, more conscious way of living. It's about understanding that every food choice you make has an impact, not just on your body, but on the world around you.

We hope that this guide has provided you with the tools and knowledge you need to successfully transition into an alkaline plant-based lifestyle. Remember, the journey toward optimal health is a marathon, not a sprint.

So, here's to you. Here's to the incredible journey you've embarked on, to the challenges you'll overcome, and to the vibrant health you're cultivating. Congratulations on taking this monumental step towards a healthier, happier, and more fulfilled life. We can't wait to see where this journey takes you.

Remember, you are not alone in this journey. You have us as your guide, and a community of fellow alkaline plant-based dieters cheering you on. We believe in you and your ability to make this positive change.

Thank you for choosing to educate yourself about this transformative lifestyle. Keep pushing forward, keep questioning, keep learning, and most importantly, keep nourishing your body with the power of alkaline, plant-based foods.

FAQ

What is an alkaline plant-based diet?

An alkaline plant-based diet focuses on the consumption of fruits, vegetables, nuts, seeds, and legumes that help to maintain the body's optimal pH level. This diet minimizes the intake of acid-forming foods such as meat, dairy, processed foods, and sugar.

How does an alkaline plant-based diet benefit my health?

By maintaining the body's optimal pH balance, an alkaline plant-based diet can potentially improve your energy levels, digestion, and immune function. It can also help with weight management and may reduce the risk of chronic diseases like diabetes, heart disease, and cancer.

Is it hard to follow an alkaline plant-based diet?

Like any lifestyle change, it can take some time to adjust to an alkaline plant-based diet. However, with a bit of planning and a focus on whole, unprocessed foods, it can be a simple and enjoyable way to eat.

Can I eat any animal products on an alkaline plant-based diet?

Animal products are generally considered acid-forming and are minimized or eliminated in an alkaline plant-based diet. However, everyone's dietary needs and preferences are different, so it's important to find a balance that works for you.

Do I need to worry about getting enough protein on an alkaline plant-based diet?

While it's a common concern, it's entirely possible to get adequate protein from plant-based sources. Foods like lentils, chickpeas, quinoa, tofu, and almonds are all high in protein.

How can I tell if my body is in an alkaline state?

You can use pH strips to test your urine or saliva to see if your body is in an alkaline state. However, these tests aren't always accurate, and it's best to focus on how you feel overall.

Are there any risks associated with an alkaline plant-based diet?

As with any diet, it's important to ensure you're getting a balanced intake of nutrients. If you're concerned about nutrient deficiencies, consider consulting with a dietitian or healthcare provider.

References and Helpful Links

Ms, J. L. (2023, November 16). The Alkaline Diet: An Evidence-Based Review. Healthline.
https://www.healthline.com/nutrition/the-alkaline-diet-myth

Lawler, M. (2024, February 14). What is the alkaline diet? review, research, alkaline food list, and more. EverydayHealth.com.
https://www.everydayhealth.com/diet-and-nutrition/diet/comprehensive-review-alkaline-diet-what-it-how-it-works-what-eat/

Acid-alkaline balance: role in chronic disease and detoxification. (2007, August 1). PubMed. https://pubmed.ncbi.nlm.nih.gov/17658124/

Blackburn, K. B. (2018, April 2). Alkaline diet: What cancer patients should know. MD Anderson Cancer Center.
https://www.mdanderson.org/cancerwise/alkaline-diet--what-cancer-patients-should-know.h00-159223356.html

Harwin, R. (2021, May 17). Benefits of an alkaline food plan in PCOS. Conquer Your PCOS Naturally.
https://www.conqueryourpcosnaturally.com/benefits-of-an-alkaline-food-plan-in-pcos/

Blackburn, K. B. (2019, May 8). The alkaline diet: What you need to know. MD Anderson Cancer Center.
https://www.mdanderson.org/publications/focused-on-health/the-alkaline-diet--what-you-need-to-know.h18-1592202.html#:~:text=The%20alkali

ne%20diet%20basically%20reinforces,alcohol%2C%20meat%20and%20processed%20foods.

Mph, E. B. (2023, August 26). Why do you need pH balance? Verywell Health. https://www.verywellhealth.com/ph-balance-significance-function-associated-conditions-5205825

Khot, M., & Khot, M. (2022, December 13). Alkaline foods – Know all about alkaline diet – Avaana. Avaana Answers. https://avaana.com.au/blog/alkaline-diet/

Alkaline diet foods, benefits, recipes and tips - Dr. Axe. (2023, May 17). Dr. Axe. https://draxe.com/nutrition/alkaline-diet/

Jędraszczyk, F., & Jędraszczyk, F. (2023, April 24). The pros and cons of following an alkaline diet. Listonic. https://listonic.com/the-pros-and-cons-of-following-an-alkaline-diet/#:~:text=One%20of%20the%20risks%20of,diet%20is%20followed%20long%2Dterm.

Research, A. I. (2024, January 7). Alkaline Diet: A Beginner's Guide and Meal Plan - Athletic Insight. Athletic Insight. https://www.athleticinsight.com/diet/alkaline

Green Scheme. (2023, December 5). Best Alkaline Recipes - Green Scheme. https://greenschemetv.net/best-alkaline-recipes/

Johnson, O. (2022, December 26). A 7-Day alkaline diet plan to rebalance PH levels and fight inflammation. BetterMe Blog. https://betterme.world/articles/7-day-alkaline-diet-plan/

Printed in the USA
CPSIA information can be obtained
at www.ICGtesting.com
CBHW070956030724
11010CB00023B/705